How to Reduce Pregnancy Stress Using the Positive Affirmations Technique

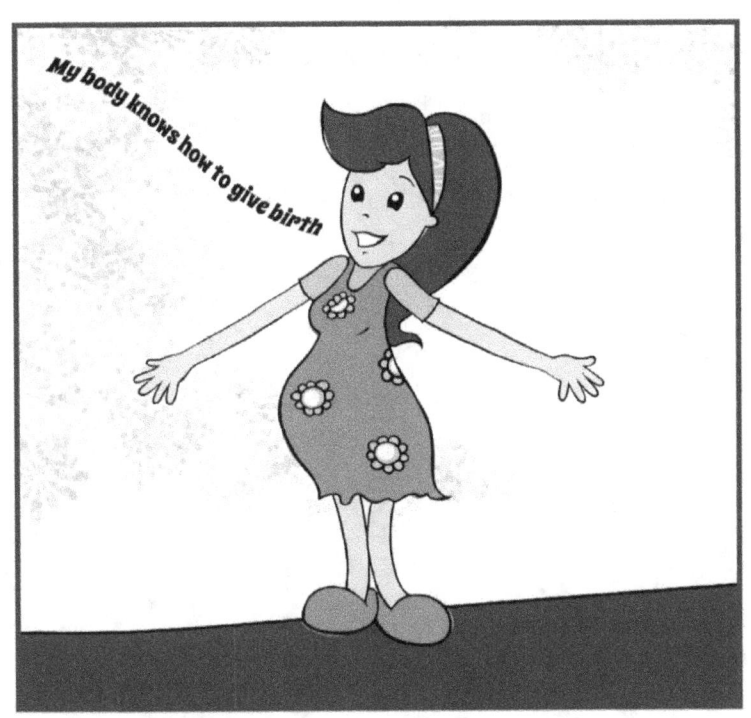

Written By: Einat L. K.

Edited By: Robert Shveytser
Book Illustrations: Leda Vaneva

How to Reduce Pregnancy Stress Using the Positive Affirmations Technique

ISBN No. 978-1630220723

First Printing, 2013

Printed in the United States of America

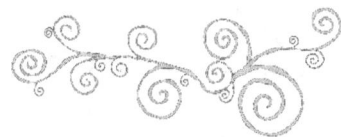

By purchasing this book you've taken the first step in minimizing your pregnancy stress and having a healthy and relaxed pregnancy for you and for your child. The next step would be to read it and use the technique it introduces. The results are sure to amaze you.

This book was written with love and care in order to support you in dealing with your pregnancy stress.

If you liked this book, please stop by and review it at:

http://www.amazon.com/dp/B00FMXCILY

Your success means a lot to me.

If you have a comment or question, please contact me at my email address:

contact@myPregnancyToolkit.com

My wish is for you to have a healthy, stress-free pregnancy accompanied by an easy, painless birth.

Scan the following code to grab a complimentary copy of your special gift for busy women. "Your Pregnancy Relaxation Kit" is designed to deal with your fears of childbirth and help you feel calmer and more relaxed during your pregnancy.

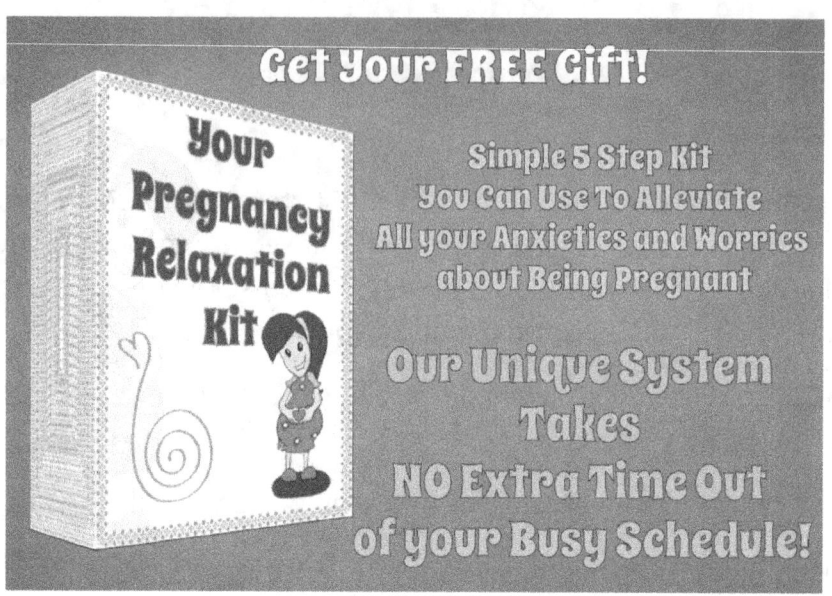

TABLE OF CONTENTS

PUBLISHER'S NOTES

Disclaimer

This publication is intended to provide the reader with helpful and informative material. It is not intended to diagnose, treat, cure, or prevent any health problem or conditions, nor is it intended to replace the advice of a physician. No medical-related action should be taken solely on the contents of this book. Always consult your physician or qualified health-care professional on any matters regarding your health and before adopting any suggestions in this book or drawing inferences from it.

The author and publisher specifically disclaim all responsibility for any liability, loss or risk, personal or otherwise, which is incurred as a consequence, directly or indirectly, from the use or application of any contents of this book.

Any and all product names referenced within this book are the trademarks of their respective owners. None of these owners have sponsored, authorized, endorsed, or approved this book.

Always read all information provided by the manufacturers' product labels before using their products. The author and publisher are not responsible for claims made by manufacturers.

Paperback Edition 2013

Manufactured in the United States of America

DEDICATION

This book is dedicated to my grandmother, who taught me to look at life with a smile on my face. No matter how stressful things get.

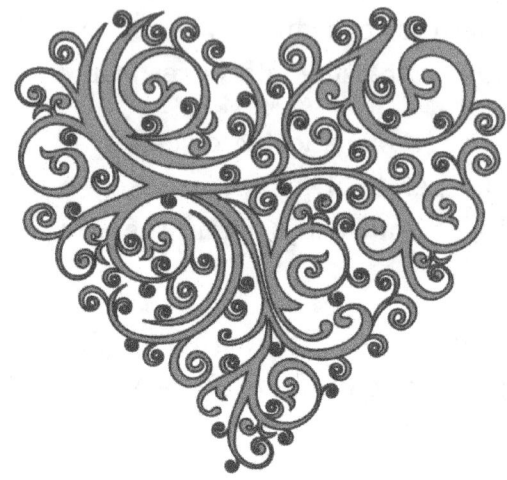

CHAPTER 1: INTRODUCTION

Greetings!

I want to congratulate you on deciding to take charge and deal with your stress during pregnancy and purchasing this book. Dealing with stress requires courage, and you show by reading this book that you have what it takes. You are a good mother to be, and your baby will benefit greatly from this decision.

This book will provide you with a technique to help you deal with stress related to pregnancy and childbirth. It will help you replace negative thoughts with positive ones, and get rid of a lot of unnecessary worries.

Pregnancy is a wonderful period in your life. It leads to the birth of your child – the amazing creation of life – which should be one of the most joyous occasions in your life. You should be happy during this period, not hung up on worries or stress.

After you have read this book you will have a great tool to deal with stress related to your pregnancy and the upcoming birth of your child. No longer will you feel frightened or stressed when you really should be calm and relaxed. You can enjoy this special period in your life and focus on yourself and your baby.

Picture yourself at the end of these nine months. You feel great; you have a smile on your face all the time. You are relaxed and you have trust in your body and in your baby. When you arrive at the hospital in time for labor, you are prepared and calm. You are full of positive thoughts and the baby is healthy and happy.

You did it! You believed in yourself, in your body and in your baby. This important time in your life passed, accompanied by happiness and tranquility. Don't forget also that the baby will feel your state of mind, and he will benefit from it as much as you do.

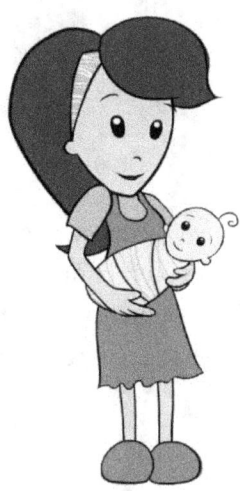

STRESS DURING PREGNANCY

Pregnancy tends to bring up a lot of buried fears to the surface. Maybe you're worried that you cannot trust your body, or that you will not be a good mother when the time arrives. All these fears cause stress, and stress can be harmful.

The definition of stress according to the Oxford dictionary is "A state of mental or emotional strain or tension resulting from adverse or demanding circumstances."

Stress is a natural part of life. Your body experiences stress as a result of various events that happen to you and your surroundings. Stress can come from your physical body, your thoughts and your surroundings. The human body is designed to experience stress and react to it. Sometimes the stress is positive when it leaves us alert and helps us avoid danger. And sometimes stress becomes negative when there is a sequence of events without any relief between them. Then the body begins to accumulate stress that can lead to trouble. Stress can affect the body in different ways: headaches, difficulty sleeping, high blood pressure, heart problems and more. When pregnant, too much stress can increase the chances of having a premature baby or a low-birth-weight baby.

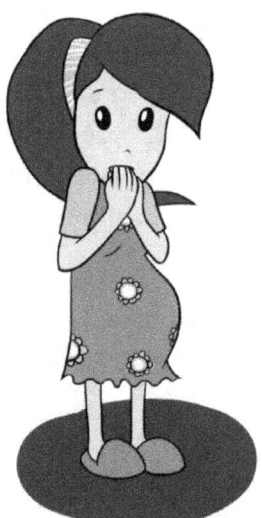

How to Reduce Stress Using the Positive Affirmations Technique will guide you in learning to release the stress and help you feel more relaxed. The technique which you will study will help bring peace and serenity into your pregnancy as well as the labor process. By reading this book you can have the calm pregnancy and relaxed childbirth that you seek.

I was in your situation when I became pregnant with my oldest daughter. At that time, I had a lot of concerns and fears, which led me to feel stressed-out most of the time. I wondered how I could ever cope and get through the pregnancy without becoming a nervous wreck. Would I *ever* feel good?

This stress had a paralyzing effect on me. I also took out my anger and frustration on my husband, friends and colleagues. Everyone told me it was the hormones, but I knew it was more than that. I feared the upcoming birth and I was afraid that the relationship with my partner would be affected. I wanted to feel better because I knew this stress wasn't good for me or the baby. It was time for me to take control and change the situation for the better.

So I began working with several tools and techniques, trying out many methods that were designed to deal with stress. In the end I found one that worked brilliantly. It helped me deal with stress in a way that no other technique could. It was easy and fun to practice, and most importantly, it showed results!

WHAT YOU CAN DO

The positive affirmation technique is a means for replacing negative thoughts with positive ones. By having a positive attitude, we can accomplish just about anything and overcome seemingly impossible obstacles.

I figured out why I was stressed, and created the special affirmations that helped me cope with and eliminate that stress. After the daily practice of these affirmations I was able to reduce my stress and bring a smile to my face on a daily basis. My friends were happy, my partner was happy and I was happy.

This book was born out of my desire to share this wonderful tool with women who have trouble dealing with stress. I know I'm not the first or last woman to find pregnancy stressful. But why should you have to go through the months of reading and researching to find methods that help you deal with your stress when I can show you this wonderful technique that will guide you in relieving your stress.

The positive affirmation technique is wonderful because it really is a tool for everyone. No matter the reason why you're stressed or how stressful your life is, you can use it to improve your situation. The technique is easy to learn and it can be practiced anywhere, anytime.

I believe that every woman deserves to have a happy pregnancy, without stress or worries. They should feel that their labor is a positive and empowering experience rather than stressful and painful. Positive affirmations are a perfect technique to use to accomplish that.

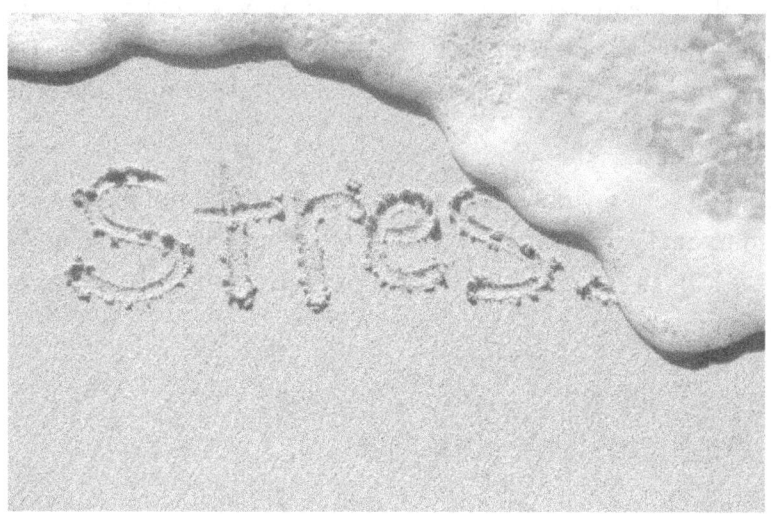

THE ROAD FROM HERE

Go ahead and jump into the water. Read the book and start to practice the exercises. Do your best and you will soon see results – a calmer, happier and safer pregnancy.

The practice only takes a few minutes of your time every day. You have several months to practice for the upcoming labor. That means you have plenty of time to work on your mind and prepare yourself for what is to come. I know that it requires some effort from you, but the rewards are great. You will be a happy, calm and relaxed mother and that will rub off on your baby.

The following chapters will discuss in detail all aspects of the Positive Affirmation tool and how to use it. Take your time, going through it. The sooner you finish, the better prepared you will be for your upcoming birth.

In order to assist you with the implementation of the technique, I invite you to download a gift – Styled Affirmations. You can print them and keep with you; hang it in a suitable corner of your room, store it in your wallet, or even choose to have it as your screensaver.

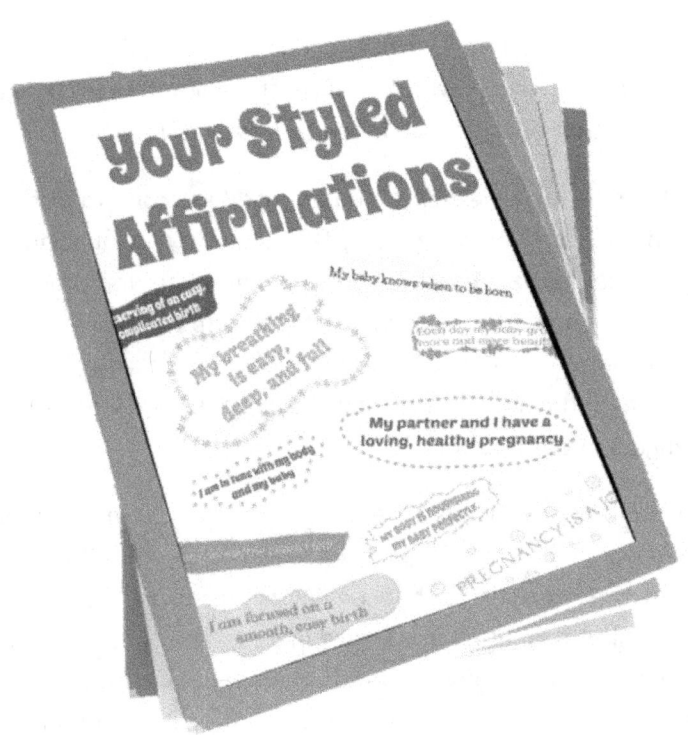

Good luck and enjoy the reading!

"If you ask me: What is the single most important key to longevity? I would have to say, it is avoiding worry, stress and tension. And if you didn't ask me, I'd still have to say it."
~ George F. Burns (comedian)

CHAPTER 2: WHAT IS AN AFFIRMATION?

WHAT ARE POSITIVE AFFIRMATIONS?

Affirmations are words or phrases which confirm that something is true or false. Positive affirmations are those that bring us into a positive state of mind.

In a way, all our thoughts are paradigms, and are used to program our subconscious. This is necessary for our survival, because by teaching our subconscious what was safe and what wasn't, we could react much faster to danger. The first time a child sees a lion and witnesses its great power, for example, she learns to think of lions as dangerous. The next time this child sees one, she could immediately run away without having to waste time wondering if the lion is dangerous. As children, we learn to react in similar ways to other dangers in our lives.

The problem is, we might not always have learned the right things and our actions as adults can be influenced by these inappropriate responses. As children, for example, we might have learned and internalized that speaking in front of others is agonizing because the other children laughed at us once in class. That doesn't mean speaking in front of other people is always going to put us in an uncomfortable or even agonizing position. Our subconscious, however, has learned that speaking to an audience is "scary", so we should stay away from it. This can cause a lot of worry and stress in children and adults.

When we were young women, we might have heard that childbirth is painful and very hard to go through. This has instilled in us the cliched belief that this is true, and our subconscious is now programmed to think of childbirth as dangerous. So, of course the thought of having to face it is stressful!

Positive affirmations are a way of changing these thought patterns. It can be thought of as brainwashing, because we wash away negative beliefs and replace them with positive ones. You are always in control of which negative beliefs you want to wash away. Through our thoughts, we can influence the way we feel. We can change our view from thinking childbirth is dangerous, for example, to thinking of it as it truly is—a remarkable and empowering experience.

THE ORIGINS OF POSITIVE AFFIRMATIONS

Positive affirmations in the form of mantras have been around in the world for centuries and are common in many Eastern religions. A mantra is a phrase or a word that can change the way people think or feel about something.

Positive affirmations have later become popular, thanks to the book (and later a film) *The Secret* by Rhonda Byrne. She, in turn, was inspired by a book from 1910 called *The Science of Getting Rich* by Wallace D. Wattles, a member of the New Thought Movement, which says that "right" thinking has a healing effect. In his book, Wattles explains how people can overcome their own barriers and attract wealth.

Other books inspired by Wattles' work are the Law of Attraction series. The law of attraction says that "like attracts like" so that a focus on positive thoughts can bring positive outcomes. By the same rule, negative thoughts can bring negative outcomes.

The effect of positive affirmations has recently been supported by scientists. Neuro-scientists have discovered that you can improve your health by changing your thoughts and incorporating more positive thinking. Thoughts create chemicals, and according to Dr. Joseph Dispenza, by changing our thoughts, we can alter that chemical compound and therefore make positive changes to our health.

Dr. Caroline Leaf, who has over 25 years of experience studying the mind and brain, says that many illnesses plaguing us today are caused by negative thinking. Fear triggers more than 1,400 physical and chemical responses, and it can activate up to 30 different hormones in our body. By constantly worrying, we gather up toxic waste which can lead to illnesses as diverse as diabetes, asthma and can even cause allergies. Cathy Chapman, a licensed clinical social worker, says that negative thoughts weaken our immune system. Replacing our "negative" thoughts with "positive" ones, is therefore important for both our mental and physical well being.

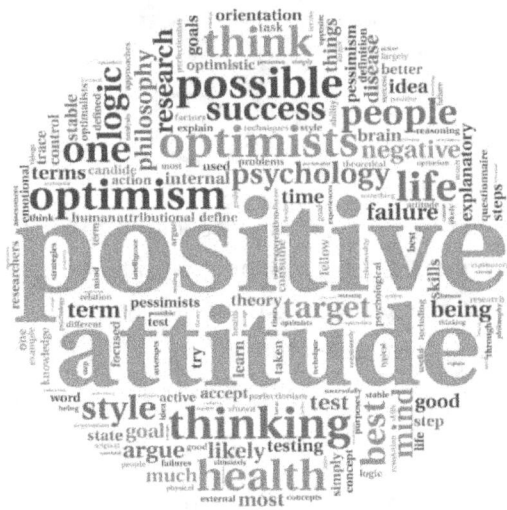

HOW DO THE POSITIVE AFFIRMATIONS WORK?

Positive affirmations force your subconscious mind to accept new, positive responses to outside influences. By constantly thinking that something is in fact not dangerous or stressful, you can convince your subconscious mind to accept that, as the new truth.

If there is a large gap between your positive affirmation and what you believe is true, you might struggle at first to get your subconscious to accept the new thoughts. Because of that, it is important to constantly practice and repeat positive affirmations.

However, if you keep repeating your positive affirmations, you will eventually manage to overcome even the fiercest resistance and change your thought patterns. Eventually, your mind will be reprogrammed so that it will accept a new truth and discard the old one.

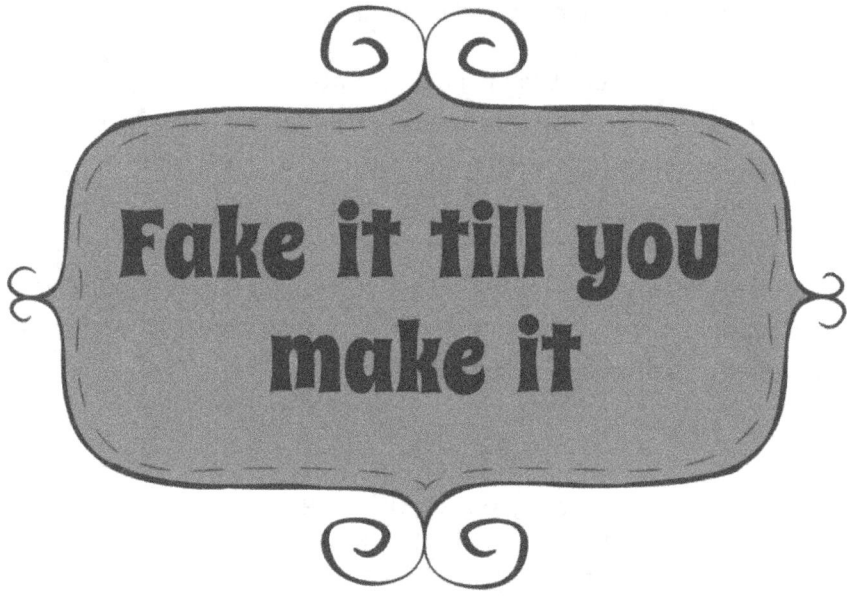

Taking an example from above, you can convince your mind that speaking in front of an audience is neither dangerous, nor stressful or agonizing. At first, you might find this hard to believe–after all, you've known the opposite to be true for a long time. Eventually however, you will start to see the effects of positive affirmations and realize that speaking before an audience actually can't hurt you. In fact, it can even be a positive experience.

The same goes for pregnancy and childbirth. No matter the reason why you are stressed during your pregnancy – if it's fear of being pregnant, of childbirth or the parenting that comes afterwards – you can reprogram your mind into thinking it is not dangerous, and there's no reason for stress or worries. Then you can finally enjoy your pregnancy the way you should.

◎ ◎ ◎ ◎ ◎ ◎ ◎

Lilly had an overpowering fear of childbirth when she was pregnant with her first child. All of her life she had heard, especially from her mother, stories about how painful and difficult it was. At first she wondered how she could ever manage to go through with it, and she was even considering a Caesarean section to avoid the stress of labor.

Then she began working with positive affirmations, and told herself every day that childbirth wasn't so bad. At first she found it difficult to believe, but eventually her mind accepted the idea and she was no longer frightened. When the time came for her labor, she was calm, relaxed and able to have a natural childbirth.

◎ ◎ ◎ ◎ ◎ ◎ ◎

In this chapter we learned about:

1. Positive affirmations and what they are

2. The history behind positive affirmations

3. How positive affirmations work

In the next chapter we will look at how positive affirmations can help reduce your stress during pregnancy.

"You become what you think about"

~ Earl Nightingale (American motivational speaker and author)

CHAPTER 3: HOW CAN POSITIVE AFFIRMATIONS HELP YOU DURING PREGNANCY AND LABOR?

THE DETRIMENTAL EFFECT OF STRESS DURING PREGNANCY

Many women feel stressed-out during their pregnancy. Your body is changing rapidly and you might be constantly worrying about the health of your child. It is completely normal, but if it causes problems during your day-to-day activities you should try to find a way to handle it.

You could also be experiencing some of the more common pregnancy problems such as morning sickness, constipation, backaches or SPD (Symphysis Pubis Dysfunction). Mood swings can be difficult for both you and your partner, and you might find that they make situations much more difficult to handle. While pregnant, you are told not to eat or drink certain things, and even what kind of exercise you can do. This puts a lot of pressure on you.

Many women are worried about the labor process. Fear of childbirth is common and can cause a lot of stress during pregnancy. You may possibly also be worried about the time that comes afterwards, about not being able to cope with having a baby, about being a bad mother or about not being able to handle the increased responsibilities.

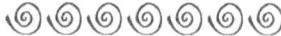

Roxanne was very stressed during her pregnancy. Combining a stressful job with all the changes in her body was very difficult for her. She also developed SPD, which meant she couldn't exercise the way she was used to. To her, walking has always been a form of relaxation and now that she wasn't able to walk for long periods of time, her blood pressure began to rise and she began having headaches.

When it was time for labor, she was so stressed that her body became very tense. Her midwife told her she needed to relax or risk that the contractions would stop altogether. That could lead to a Caesarean section. Finally, she was able to calm herself down. She had a natural childbirth, but she knew she had been very close to a C-section just because she was so stressed.

HOW TO TREAT STRESS IN A NATURAL WAY WITHOUT MEDICATION

There are plenty of good ways to deal with your stress. Start saying *no* to tasks, at work or at home which make you feel stressful. Cut down on your chores and make sure you get enough time to relax. Learn to ask for help from friends, family or your partner. Take some time to simply sit down, take a nap or read a book.

You need to get exercise: walking or swimming is great. Relaxing exercises like yoga, stretching or Pilates might also help you through this time. Eating a healthy diet can give you an extra energy boost, and it can even reduce your stress levels. That's one reason why it's so important to eat nutritious food during your pregnancy.

When you do run out of energy, make sure to go to bed for a full night's sleep. You will require more sleep than usual during your pregnancy, so make sure you go to bed early, so that you're well-rested in the morning.

One of the most useful and easiest tools to use to reduce your stress is positive affirmations. Positive affirmations can be combined with the Image Visualization Technique, which is another valuable tool for reducing stress. This technique is similar to positive affirmations, but it's based more on images than words. It includes focusing on positive images of the future, in your mind or on a vision board.

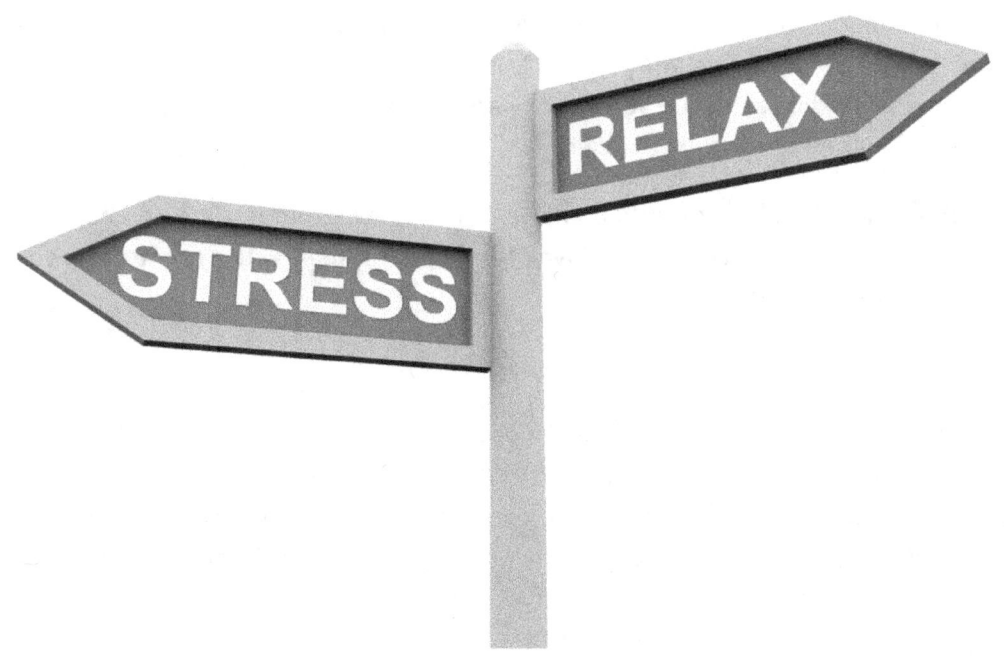

JUST HOW POSITIVE IS A POSITIVE AFFIRMATION FOR A PREGNANT WOMAN?

By repeating positive words or statements, you can change the way you think about something, from negatively to positively. That is a very valuable tool for stress reduction.

If you feel worried throughout your pregnancy about the health of your baby, you can use positive affirmations to reprogram your mind from constant worry, to confidence in yourself and the future. Use positive affirmations to turn stress regarding your changing body into excitement about this stage in your life.

Instead of seeing the common pregnancy symptoms such as nausea and SPD as problems, use positive affirmations to see them as signs of what your body is capable of accomplishing. Positive affirmations can make you strong, and confident in your body's ability to create and give birth to a new life. They will keep you from worrying too much and help calm you down...

Many women fear the stages of labor, from being able to cope with the pain, to the effects childbirth will have on their body afterwards. If you are constantly stressed about the pain you think you will feel, use positive affirmations to remind yourself that this is what your body was made for. Positive affirmations can calm your nerves when you're concerned about having a child pass through your vagina, and it can reduce your worries about vaginal tearing.

If you are primarily worried about what comes after childbirth or about not being able to cope as a mother, positive affirmations are an effective way to give yourself confidence. With this technique you can replace the fear of failing as a mother with confidence in your own natural abilities.

No matter which stage of motherhood may worry you: whether it is the pregnancy, childbirth or the time afterwards, *positive affirmations* is an effective tool to help you turn stress into calm confidence.

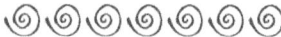

Johanna was very stressed even before she became pregnant with her first child, and when she was pregnant she found she wasn't able to take it any longer. She constantly worried about the health of her baby, her job, and about becoming a parent. When her doctor told her she had high blood pressure (in her first trimester), she realized she had to do something about it.

Johanna learned everything she could about positive affirmations and she began implementing it in her own life. Now she was feeling much calmer and more relaxed. Her blood pressure went down, and she eventually experienced a healthy and happy pregnancy. After the birth of her daughter, she also found that positive affirmations could help her become a better mother. She was still relaxed and calm even when her baby developed colic, confident in the knowledge that the condition would pass. When she returned to work, she found that she was much more relaxed, as well.

⊚ ⊚ ⊚ ⊚ ⊚ ⊚ ⊚

In this chapter you learned about:

1. Stress during pregnancy

2. Tools for dealing with stress

3. Positive affirmations and stress

In the next chapter we will learn about the effects of stress on your growing baby and the importance of reducing it in your life.

"There must be quite a few things that a hot bath won't cure, but I don't know many of them."

~Sylvia Plath (poet)

CHAPTER 4: WHAT IS THE EFFECT OF THE POSITIVE AFFIRMATION ON YOUR FETUS?

THE EFFECTS OF STRESS ON YOUR BABY

Stress is a normal part of life and our bodies cope with it every day. Stress has many negative effects on your body, and you might not even be aware that stress is the cause. It can cause tension, headaches and muscle pains, as well as upset stomach or sleepless nights. In some cases, stress can even lead to depression.

Your baby is very vulnerable during his time in your uterus and can be affected by your state of mind. Too much stress may damage your immune system, which could lead to infections. If you suffer from a severe infection, your baby's health might be in danger and it could trigger a premature birth.

Stress can cause the production of a hormone known as corticotrophin (CRH), which is also produced naturally by the body to trigger contractions. Scientists believe that this could be the reason why stress increases the risk of preterm labor. Children born before they are due are not fully developed, and they are more likely to suffer from problems such as infections, jaundice and cerebral palsy.

Miscarriage is one of the worst things that can happen, and most often it is caused by fetal abnormalities. However, studies have found a link between stress and a high risk of miscarriage. This is especially the case just after conception or in the early stages of pregnancy. Studies have suggested that the stress hormone CRH can lead to a disruption of the placenta and thus prevent the embryo from developing properly.

Many hormones linked to stress can cause your blood vessels to constrict, preventing nutrients to pass from you to your baby. That is why stress is often linked to low birth weight. Not all children born with a low birth weight suffer from it, but some might have problems with low blood sugar and other birth defects.

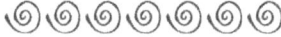

Lindsey suffered from severe stress when she was pregnant with her first child because her mother had recently died from a heart attack. Lindsey was only a few weeks pregnant when she suffered a miscarriage, which according to her doctors could have been caused by the stress brought on by the grief she was experiencing.

◎ ◎ ◎ ◎ ◎ ◎ ◎

HOW YOUR STATE OF MIND AFFECTS YOUR BABY

Studies have shown that your baby's later development is influenced by your state of mind during the pregnancy. In cases where the mother was stressed out, children have been more at risk of developmental, emotional or physical problems. These effects might not be apparent at first, but they can influence the child later in life.

The child's physical development is strongly affected by the state of your emotional being and mental health during your pregnancy. Studies have shown that children born to stressed-out mothers are more at risk of diabetes and obesity than those whose mothers were calm and relaxed.

According to the studies, the mother's emotional state during pregnancy can affect the genetics of the baby. This means that a stressed-out mother is more likely to give birth to a child who may develop problems down the line, due to his or her own nervousness or anxiety. When the situation is reversed, a happy mother should be more likely to give birth to a happy and calm child. As you can see, your baby can only benefit from your dealing with your your stress and becoming more relaxed.

According to Curt A. Sandman, who researched how the mother's state of mind affects the baby, your baby is collecting information for how its life will be after birth. "It's preparing for life based on messages the mom is providing," he says. By having a happy and calm pregnancy, you are teaching your baby that that is how his life will be in the future.

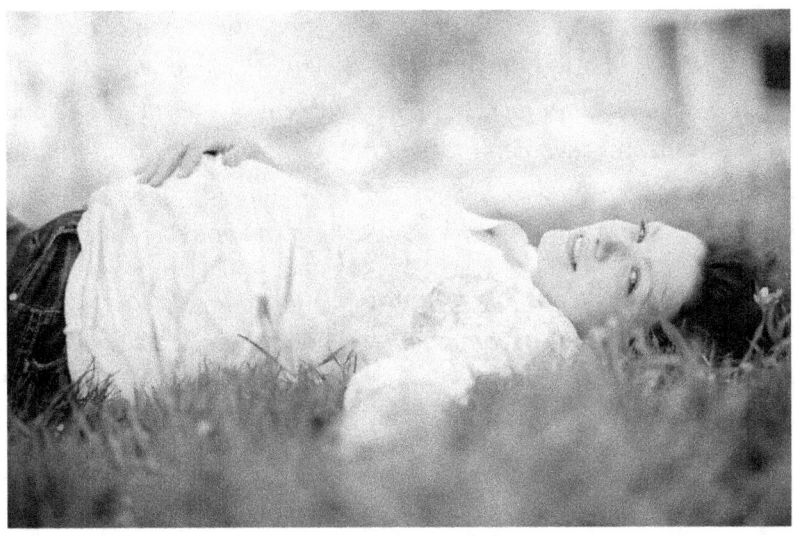

THE EFFECTS OF POSITIVE AFFIRMATIONS ON YOUR BABY

Now that your baby is developing his body and mind that he will live with for the rest of his life, he is very influenced by your emotions. By taking care of yourself and avoiding stress, you can begin providing a better environment for your baby. Not only will you be reducing the risks of a miscarriage or premature birth, but you'll also be increasing his chances to be born happy and healthy.

All our thoughts come with emotions, and negative thoughts bring negative emotions into our lives. Your baby can feel these emotions and become affected by them. If you could change your negative (or damaging) thoughts into positive ones, your baby would feel the difference. Practicing positive affirmations is a way of training your mind to think positively, and you can start to train your baby to think positive thoughts by doing so yourself. That will give your child a great start in life.

When you focus your positive affirmations on gaining confidence during pregnancy, your baby will gain confidence too. The chemicals passing through the placenta will make him calm and self-assured. Remember that you're teaching him that you are a confident mother and that he can rely on you no matter what. He will know that when he is born, and his life will be relaxed and happy without fears or worries.

A mother who practices the positive affirmations technique will be more relaxed and able to deal with uncertainties. That means you will perform even better as a mother and will be able to take care of your baby the way you want.

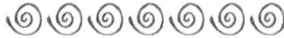

Mary was stressed during the first half of her pregnancy, worrying about how life would be like now that she was about to have a child. Her relationship with the baby's father was unstable for a while, further increasing her worries for the future. A sonogram during her second trimester revealed that her baby was not developing as she should. Mary's doctor thought this could be because Mary wasn't eating enough, and that her stress was reducing the amount of nutrients reaching the baby.

Mary began working with the positive affirmations technique as soon as she found out about it and found that she was becoming happier and more relaxed. Her daughter was only slightly underweight when born and had no complications due to this. Mary used her positive affirmations to reunite with the baby's father and live a more stress-free life afterwards.

In this chapter you learned about:

1. The effects of stress on your baby

2. How your state of mind affects your baby

3. The effects of positive affirmations on your baby

In the next chapter we will be looking at how to make your own positive affirmations and how you can use them.

"Before you were conceived I wanted you. Before you were born I loved you. Before you were here an hour I would die for you. This is the miracle of Mother's Love"

~ Maureen Hawkins (author)

CHAPTER 5: HOW TO BUILD YOUR OWN AFFIRMATION

HOW TO CHOOSE YOUR AFFIRMATIONS

Positive affirmations only work if they ring true to you and your specific needs. If we feel like we are lying to ourselves, our subconscious won't be as easy to convince that we feel our affirmation is right. Affirmations are very personal and should put you in focus. That's why an affirmation that you've written yourself might work better than using someone else's.

Looking at other people's positive affirmations can inspire you and let you know what kind of affirmation you want for yourself. Because of that, you shouldn't feel nervous about looking at affirmations online or in magazines. Once you begin working with positive affirmations however, it is always best to write your own.

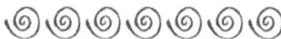

Britney wanted to work with positive affirmations, but she didn't know how. She found some affirmations online and began repeating them every day. However, she never felt that the affirmations rang true. After weeks of repeating them, she still wondered why her state of mind hadn't changed.

A friend told her about the value of creating your own positive affirmations. Britney sat down one evening and rephrased the affirmations she had been using so they would feel more personal. Now she began seeing results very quickly, and she was able to transform her state of mind. The most stressful issue she had was that she was nervous that the baby is not ok and not healthy. She created her affirmation to say: "My baby is healthy and happy".

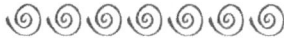

SIMPLE, EASY STEPS TO CREATE YOUR OWN AFFIRMATIONS

Creating your own positive affirmations is simple, and all you have to do is follow these steps:

Step 1 - Find a quiet place:

 Sit down in a quiet place. Make yourself comfortable.

Step 2 - Find your stressful issues:

 Think about why you're feeling stressed out. What causes stress in your life?

Write down 5 causes of stress during your pregnancy. You can download the practice worksheet from the following qrcode.

Your Practice Worksheet

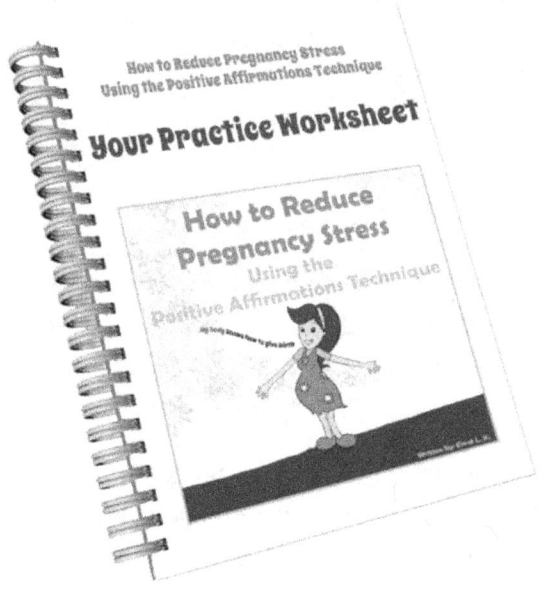

To give you an example, my 5 most stressful issues were:

- I'm afraid my body won't come back to normal after childbirth

- I'm afraid of the stage where the child passes through my vagina

- I'm petrified when I think about the labor process

- I'm so stressed at work that I can't calm down

- I'm afraid my baby won't be born healthy

Step 3 - Find your restrictive beliefs:

For each item on the list, ask yourself, what's behind the stressful issue? What do you think is causing this stress? As these ideas and thoughts come to you, think about your personality traits and how stress affects you specifically.

For example, when I used to worry that my body wouldn't return to normal, I always felt like I was fat. When I worried about the child passing through my vagina, I always felt that my muscles around my vagina were tight and clenched. That was the person I was when I worried about these things.

These are your "restrictive beliefs", or the ideas that are currently holding you back.

Step 4 - Create your positive affirmation:

Now that you've spotted your restrictive beliefs, you are ready to create your own affirmation. What you need to do is think about what you can say to yourself to neutralize the influence of your restrictive belief. What can you say that will change your mind?

For example, when I felt I was fat and was worried about my body not returning to normal, I could neutralize my state of mind by thinking I was beautiful. When I worried about the child passing through my vagina, I needed to know I was open and flexible.

Write down a sentence for each of the 5 negative beliefs that will describe this neutralization as accurately as possible. Write it in the present tense and don't include words like "wish" or "would". This is extremely important; you are already what you want to be, right now. The subconscious knows only the present tense. The sentence should describe a positive state you wish to be in, but in present tense.

Make your affirmations positive. Avoid using negative words like pain, stress, worry. Instead, replace them with words like health, calm, relaxation. Don't write, "I am not in pain", but instead, "I am healthy."

Your affirmations work best if they are short and simple. That way you don't have to memorize anything and you can repeat your affirmations as many times as you want throughout the day. Be specific about what you want and describe and the state of mind in which you want to b.

Step 5 - Utilize your affirmation:

Congratulations, you now have 5 positive affirmations that can be utilized to reduce your stress levels.

Step 6 - Shortcut - use pre-made affirmations:

If you found that this process was difficult or didn't work for you, feel free to use instead, some of the positive affirmations I suggest in the coming chapters. There is nothing wrong with using pre-made positive affirmations as long as they work for you, and you can use as many affirmations as you want.

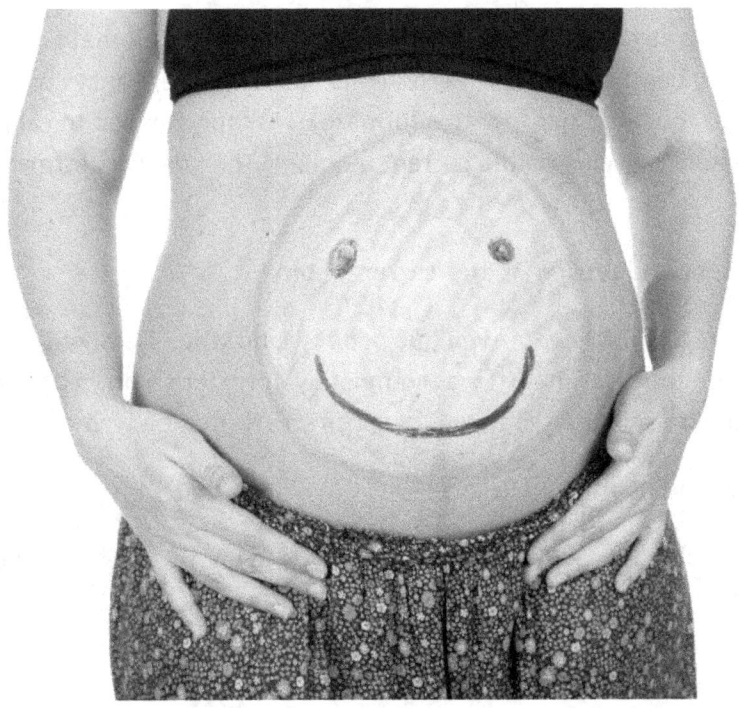

A PRACTICAL EXAMPLE

After I had specified my own five causes of stress during pregnancy, I sat down and went through the steps above. For the first one – *I'm afraid my body won't come back to normal after childbirth* – I found that my restrictive belief was that I thought I was physically unattractive. In order to neutralize that state of mind, I needed to feel that I was beautiful. My positive affirmation became:

- I am beautiful.

For my second concern, *I'm afraid of the stage where the child passes through my vagina*, I felt tight and clenched. In order to neutralize that feeling, I needed to feel relaxed and ready. My affirmation therefore became:

- I am relaxed and ready to give birth to my child.

The third one was *I'm petrified when I think about the labor*. When that thought came to my mind, I was afraid and became very stressed-out. In order to neutralize it, I needed to feel empowered.

- I am strong.

When I thought *I'm so stressed at work that I can't calm down*, I felt that I can't focus on my work because my head was filled with thoughts about my pregnancy checks and all the preparations for the birth. In order to neutralize it, I simply needed to calm down by believing in myself and focusing on the current moment. The positive affirmation I wrote was:

- I am calm, confident and present in this current moment.

The last one was, *I'm afraid my baby won't be healthy,* and when I thought it, I was always worried. Even though I knew it was completely normal to worry about the health of my child, I needed to calm myself down. My positive affirmation was:

- My baby is happy and healthy.

These affirmations helped me a lot during pregnancy, and I hope you can be helped too by creating your own affirmations.

In this chapter you learned about:

1. How to choose your affirmations

2. Creating your own affirmations

3. You've seen some practical examples

In the next chapter we will have a look at how you should use your positive affirmations for the best results.

"Most people live, whether physically, intellectually or morally, in a very restricted circle of their potential being. They make very small use of their possible consciousness and of their soul's resources in general, much like a man who, out of his whole bodily organism, should get into a habit of using and moving only his little finger."

~William James (philosopher)

CHAPTER 6: HOW TO USE YOUR AFFIRMATION

HOW TO USE YOUR AFFIRMATIONS

Now that you have written your affirmations, the real work of using them can begin. Until now, the sentences were just words written down on paper with little power to change your mind about pregnancy and stress. But *now* is when you can begin the most important part of the process: using your positive affirmations.

As you already know from previous chapters, affirmations work because they have the power to change your subconscious' response to certain things. A stressful response to the thought of childbirth can be changed into one of calm and anticipation, for example.

The only way positive affirmations can work is by becoming completely embedded into your mind, where they can change your subconscious. Only then can they begin to take effect, reducing your stress and making you feel calmer and more relaxed. That's the time when you'll start feeling better about your pregnancy and it will benefit both you and your baby.

REPETITION FOR BEST EFFECT

The key to using positive affirmations is repetition. Only by repeating your affirmation often and regularly can it become a part of your subconscious and change the way you think, feel and respond to thoughts. Below is a step-by-step guide to how you should work with your positive affirmations for the best result.

Step 1:

Choose one of the affirmations on your list with which you will begin. You can do so with the one that gives you most stress, if you want. The important thing is for you to choose one that you feel is right and would want to use to start.

Choosing only one affirmation to begin with allows you to focus on embedding one thought into your subconscious fully before moving on to the next. It also makes it *easier* for you, since you only have to memorize one affirmation at a time and fully focus on it.

Step 2:

For 21 days you should do the following:

- Pick times to work on your affirmations during the day. You can decide to work on them in the morning or in the evening, whichever suits you best. Get into the habit of repeating the affirmations daily.

- Have a notebook and pen dedicated to your affirmations. Write the affirmation down 10 times in your notebook.

- Smile to yourself and repeat the affirmation in front of a mirror.

- Repeat the positive affirmation to yourself as often as possible during the day. It can be in your car while driving to work, while you're taking a shower or while you're doing the laundry.

- You can also make a recording of your positive affirmation and listen to it.

- You can choose a time of day when you can relax, sit down, listen to some good music and repeat your positive affirmation.

- Keep the affirmation within your sight during the whole day: Use the positive affirmation as a screen saver and write it as a reminder in your cell phone. Print the affirmation and hang it around the house or in your office. You can also keep it in your wallet.

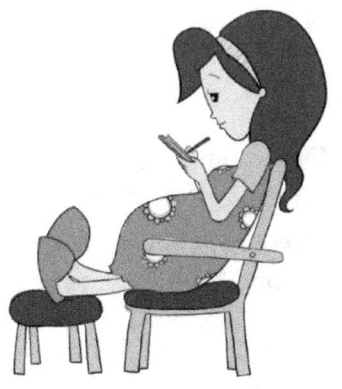

Step 3:

At the end of these 21 days (as a rule of thumb), the affirmation should be a part of you. Sit down and reflect on how different you feel and how your stress is reduced. You probably still have a few more affirmations to go, so don't worry if you're not already feeling completely calm. However, you should feel that the stress is reduced when it comes to the particular problem related to your first affirmation.

If you want to, you can record in a diary how different you feel about the subject that worried you. That way, you will notice steady improvements in your stress. Often it's difficult to notice changes when they happen over a long period of time, because we become so used to them. That's why it's good to have a record of how you felt before you started working with your positive affirmation, and of how you're feeling now.

Step 4:

If you forget to use your positive affirmation one day, start the whole process of embedding the affirmation into your subconscious from the beginning. You don't need to rush these things, but let them take as much time as you need. If you find it difficult to remember to work on your affirmations, look over your routine and try to find a way to include them. Put a reminder somewhere it will be visible, such as on your refrigerator or beside your bed.

Step 5:

Once an affirmation is embedded in your subconscious, you are ready to move on to the next one. If you still feel, after 21 days, that you would like to take some more time working on your affirmation, do so. The point is not to stress about anything, so don't worry about working with your affirmations! It should be a positive, relaxing experience and you move on to your next positive affirmation when you are ready.

Step 6:

In order to keep the old affirmations embedded in your subconscious, repeat them once a week. Set some time apart to work on all your affirmations, so they will stay fresh in your mind. You might also want to set up reminders or pin posters around your house to remind you of these affirmations.

HOW AFFIRMATIONS REDUCE YOUR STRESS

As mentioned earlier, you should soon start to feel more relaxed and at peace. The stress will go away and you will have programmed your own mind into thinking positive thoughts instead of negative ones.

ⓖ ⓖ ⓖ ⓖ ⓖ ⓖ ⓖ

Laura was very stressed during her pregnancy and found it very difficult to relax. She began working with positive affirmations, but at first she found it stressful to have to remember to actually work on them every day. So she put up an inspirational poster beside her bed.

Now that this inspirational poster was the first thing she saw every morning, instead of snoozing and fretting about all she had to do during the day–as she usually did in the morning–she began repeating the positive affirmations to herself. Eventually it became a part of her morning routine. Every Saturday she would repeat all of her previous affirmations, and she began to feel a significant change in her entire body and mind. Now her mornings were no longer stressful.

ⓖ ⓖ ⓖ ⓖ ⓖ ⓖ ⓖ

In this chapter you learned about:

1. How to use your affirmations

2. How repetition is used for best effect

3. How affirmations reduce your stress

In the next chapter, we will look at a shortcut to creating and using positive affirmations for the busy woman with little time on her hands.

"Don't wait. The time will never be just right."

~Napoleon Hill (American author)

CHAPTER 7: YOUR PRE-MADE AFFIRMATIONS – A SHORTCUT FOR CREATING YOUR AFFIRMATIONS

WHY USE A SHORTCUT

Some women find it hard to sit down and create their own affirmations. They might not have the time or energy to go through the process of thinking through their worries and stress. Some might find the process itself very stressful and prefer to begin with an affirmation already created by someone else. Or they could find it difficult to put their finger on what's really stressing them out.

If this sounds like you, don't worry. Positive affirmations are very efficient tools for dealing with stress regardless of whether you've made your own affirmation or if you're using one made by someone else. As long as you feel that the affirmation works for you and rings true to what you want to accomplish, do what you think is best.

$$\circledcirc \; \circledcirc \; \circledcirc \; \circledcirc \; \circledcirc \; \circledcirc \; \circledcirc$$

Cynthia wasn't able to write her own positive affirmations because she always felt there was something in the way. Before her pregnancy and during her first trimester she was very busy with work and never seemed to have enough time to write her own affirmations. At first she thought she should give up on the idea, until she decided to begin with pre-made affirmations.

Now she was able to immediately begin working on her own stress. She found one that felt right for her and worked with that positive affirmation according to the instructions she had received. Only a few weeks later she could already tell that her stress was reduced. When it was time for her child to be born, she was a much more relaxed person.

$$\circledcirc \; \circledcirc \; \circledcirc \; \circledcirc \; \circledcirc \; \circledcirc \; \circledcirc$$

COMMON CAUSES FOR STRESS DURING PREGNANCY

There are many reasons to feel stress during pregnancy. Here are the most common issues and fears women experience while they are pregnant.

- **Fear that the body won't return to normal after pregnancy.** It is common to worry about how your body will look after your pregnancy, but through positive affirmations you can turn that worry into self-confidence.

- **Fear that you may do something that hurts the baby.** Worrying about eating something you shouldn't or sleeping on your stomach, and thus harming your baby, is common. Positive affirmations are a great way to deal with this fear.

 - **Fear of pain.** Many women associate childbirth with pain, but you *can* change the way you think about it, to see childbirth as a wonderful and empowering experience.

- **Fear of your baby passing through your vagina.** There may be tearing and bruising when the baby passes through the vagina, and sometimes just the thought of this stage frightens women.

- **Fear of tenseness due to pressure and stress.** Many women feel stressed-out because they can't get rid of their own stress. This can become a vicious circle. But don't worry, with positive affirmations you can work on this and start seeing improvements in no time.

- **Fear of the unknown.** First-time mothers might find it difficult to cope with the unknown aspects of pregnancy. Dealing with it can help you in the future as well, since there are many aspects of life that are unknown.

- **Fear that the labor won't proceed the way you have planned.** Many women find it difficult to be out of control, especially when it comes to labor. You can deal with this very effectively by using positive affirmations.

- **Fear of episiotomy.** During childbirth you might have to have an episiotomy, which is a controlled cut to let your baby pass through your vagina. You should remember that this is done for you and your child's benefit. Work on removing the fear with positive affirmations.

- **Fear of complications.** There is always the possibility that something will go wrong during childbirth, but worrying about it will not help you or your baby. Work on dealing with this fear and will be at the same time lowering the risks of complications due to stress and tenseness.

- **Fear of dying during childbirth.** The risk of dying during childbirth is very low, but many women still worry about it. If you suffer from this fear, make sure to work on your positive affirmations to let yourself relax.

- **Fear for the health of the baby.** Most women worry at some point during their pregnancy about the health of their child. If the stress becomes too much for you to handle however, you should work with positive affirmations and let yourself relax. Your baby will not be healthier just because you worry. In fact, the very opposite may be the case.

- **Fear that you might not be able to cope with raising a child.** Many women worry that they won't be good mothers or that they will "lose" themselves after their child is born. Positive affirmations are a great way to gain confidence in yourself and your own abilities.

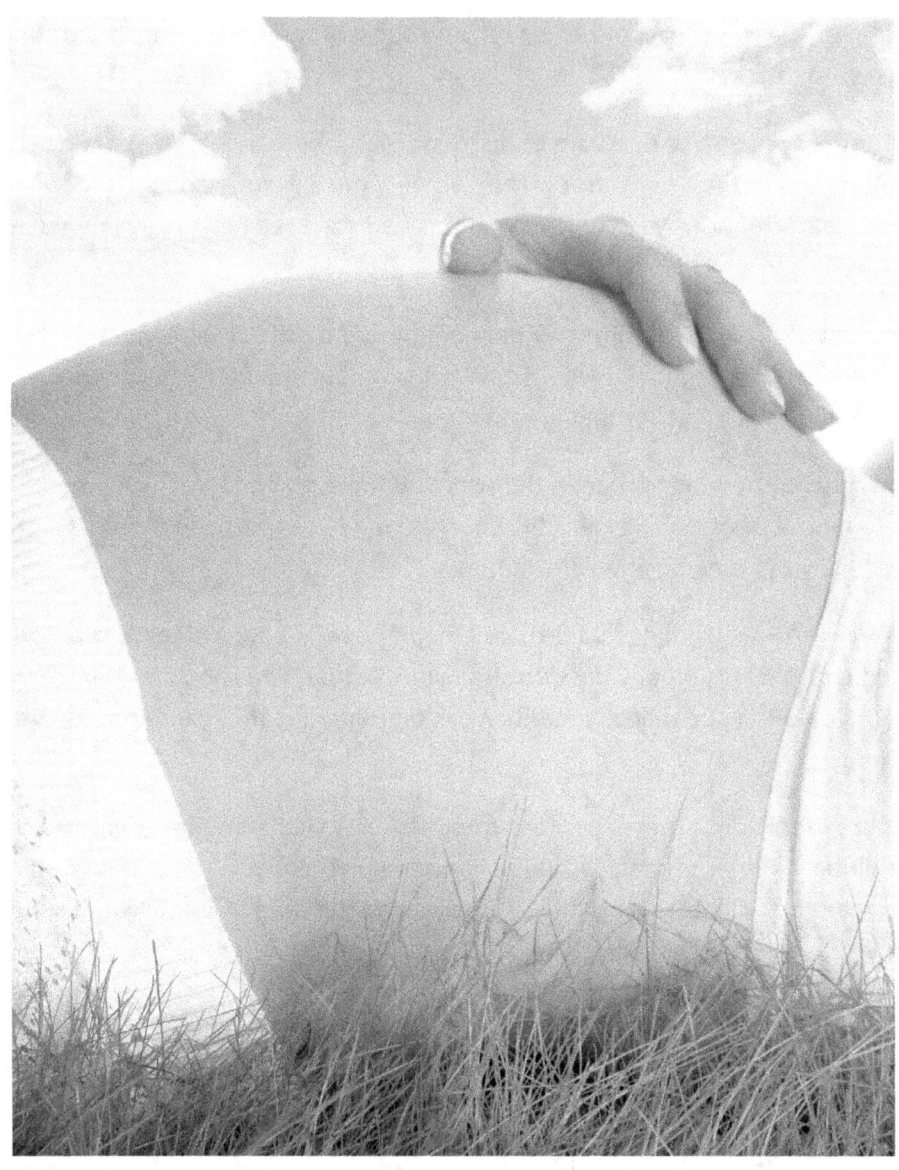

If you prefer to work with pre-made affirmations for reducing stress, you are welcome to use from the following list. Choose one that fits you personally and that you feel good about. Use it in the way described in Chapter 6.

Affirmations for the pregnancy

These affirmations are valuable for stress related to your pregnancy, your changing body and this particular period in time.

- Everything is going perfectly during my pregnancy.
- I have courage, faith and patience.
- I am in complete control of what is going on around me.
- I love my happy, healthy, pregnant body.
- Whenever I'm tired it is just a sure sign my baby is growing and developing exactly as it should do.
- I know how to take care of myself during pregnancy.
- I am a good mother.
- I am a strong woman.
- My pregnant body is beautiful.
- I accept the help of others.
- I am surrounded by those who love and respect me.
- Everything is going perfectly during my pregnancy.
- I am in complete control of what is going on around me.
- I am in tune with my body and my baby.
- I embrace my strength.
- I embrace my power.
- I surrender to my body's wisdom.
- I am fit, healthy and attractive.
- My possibilities are endless.
- I am confident.
- I have abundant energy, vitality and well-being.
- My body is beautiful, capable and strong.
- My partner and I have a loving, healthy pregnancy.
- It is safe for me to have my baby.
- I am healthy, happy and pregnant.
- My belly is full of light and love.

- I have patience.
- My baby feels my joy.
- I ask for and receive what I need.
- I am surrounded by loving, nurturing support.
- My body is nourishing my baby perfectly.
- Pregnancy is a joy.
- I am aware of my balanced, calm pregnancy.
- My body becomes stronger and more flexible every day.
- I cooperate with my body and my baby.
- I desire foods that nourish me and support my health.
- I can handle whatever comes up.
- I completely rely on my body.
- I love this pregnancy.
- This pregnancy is very special.
- I love my body.
- All is well.
- I will keep the baby safe 'till labor.

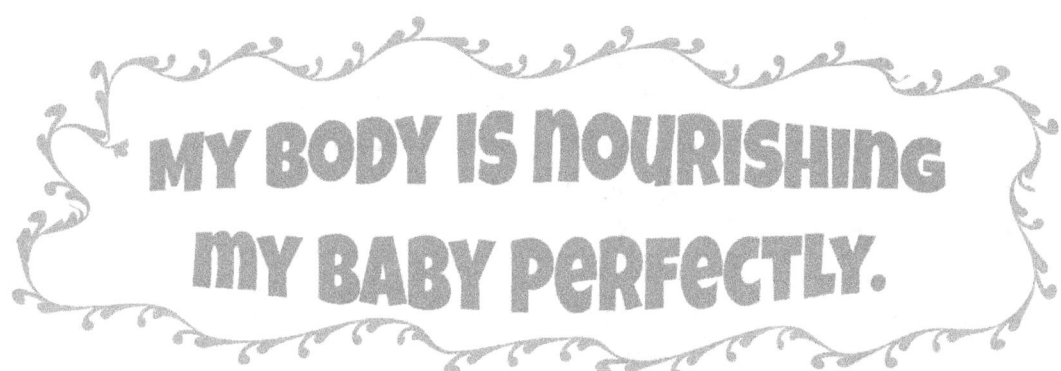

Affirmations for the baby

These affirmations can help you deal with stress and worry related to your baby, if you worry about his health or wellbeing.

- When I eat, I am feeding my baby, not myself
- My baby will find the perfect position for birth.
- I love my baby.
- My baby loves me.
- I will make the right decisions for my baby.
- My baby senses the peace I feel.
- My baby feels my love.
- I will make plenty of breast milk for my baby.
- My baby is happy and healthy
- I can do this
- I trust my body to deliver to me a healthy baby
- I welcome my baby into this world with an open heart filled with love.
- I have nothing to fear.
- I feel my baby growing inside of me.
- I am so happy that my baby is healthy and beautiful.
- Each day my baby grows more and more beautiful.
- I feel confident about my baby growing healthy and strong.
- Each day I love my baby more and more; each day brings us closer.
- My baby is strong and resilient.
- I feel my baby's peace and love.
- My baby feels my love.
- Every day my baby increase in size in a perfect way.
- I feel so comfortable having my baby with me.
- I am sending my baby comfort and love and security.
- My energy is giving my baby strength to grow healthy and wise
- My baby will be the best in the world
- I am going to have a beautiful baby
- My baby feels my calm and confidence.
- My baby knows when to be born
- My baby knows the way out

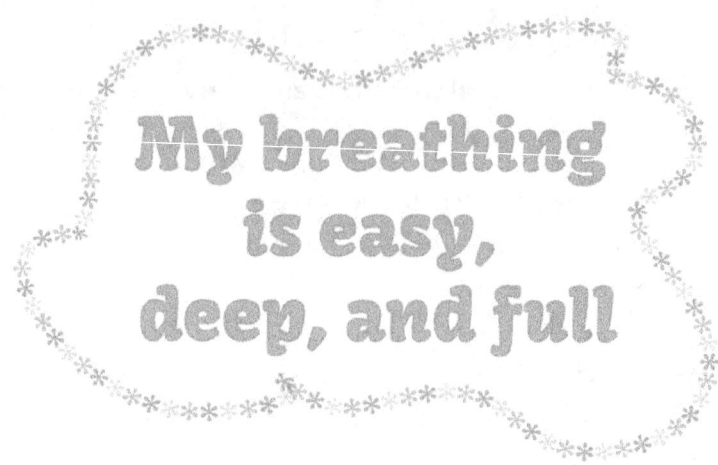

Affirmations for the labor

These affirmations are meant to help you deal with stress and fear related to the labor process, such as fear of dying or fear of the pain you might feel during childbirth.

- My body knows how to give birth.
- Birth is safe for me and my baby.
- My baby will be born at the perfect time.
- My body knows when to give birth.
- Contractions help to deliver my baby.
- I accept my labor and your birth.
- I trust my body.
- My baby will find the perfect position for birth.
- I know how to take care of my baby.
- I am excited to give birth to my baby.
- I trust in my ability to birth my baby.
- During labor and birth, I am completely relaxed.
- I am deserving of an easy, uncomplicated birth.
- I visualize my baby moving gently through the birth canal.
- I visualize an easy, peaceful, joyous and pleasurable birth.
- I am completely cooperating with my body.
- My courage and patience will send my baby into my arms.
- My body is made to give birth, nice and easy.
- My body is completely relaxed.

- I do not fight the birth in any way. My body is relaxed.
- I am a birth warrior.
- I put all fear aside as I prepare for the birth of my baby.
- I am relaxed, and happy that my baby is finally coming to me.
- My baby is free to choose her own destiny in the world.
- I am focused on a smooth, easy birth.
- I feel confident; I feel safe; I feel secure.
- I welcome this opportunity to grow and change.
- My cervix opens outward and allows my baby to ease down.
- I fully relax and turn my birthing over to Nature.
- I turn my birthing over to my baby and my body.
- I am willing to release my baby into the world.
- My baby's birth will be easy because I am so relaxed.
- My breathing is easy, deep, and full.
- I trust my intuition.
- I put all fear aside and welcome by baby with happiness and joy.
- My mind and muscles are relaxed.
- My body has a wide open space for my baby to descend.
- I am perfectly designed for labor.
- I have the energy and stamina to birth my baby.
- I allow my body's natural anesthesia to flow through my body.
- I can handle contractions.
- I can manage all pain.

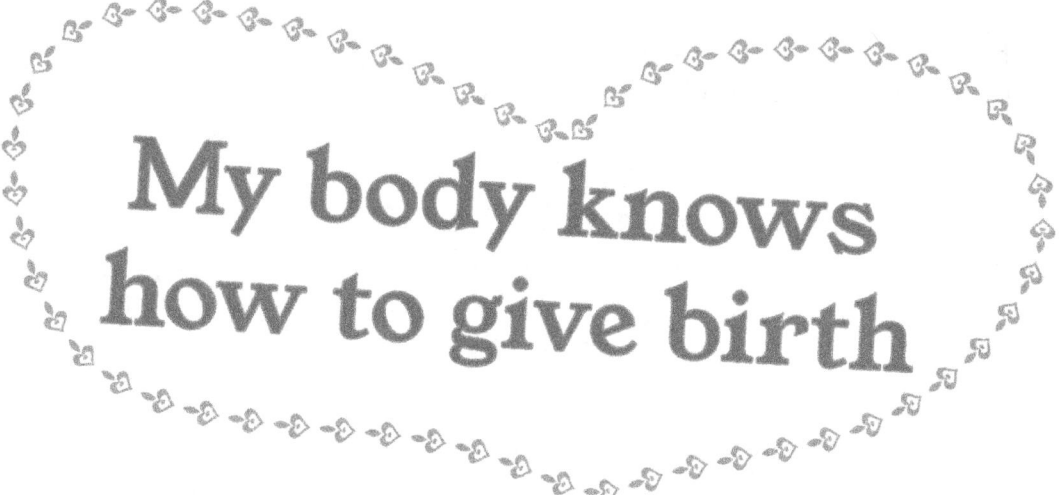

◎ ◎ ◎ ◎ ◎ ◎ ◎

Harriet was very stressed during her pregnancy and she could tell it wasn't just because of her hormones. She constantly felt tense and uneasy, but had no real worries to put her finger on. When she began working with positive affirmations, she found it difficult to write down her restrictive beliefs.

Eventually she decided to give up the thought of positive affirmations altogether, thinking it probably wasn't for her. She was still stressed-out, and no matter how hard she tried she never managed to calm down and relax. When she entered her second trimester however, she realized she needed a change, or she would risk high blood pressure as a result.

Harriet went on to use a pre-made pregnancy affirmation. It turned out this affirmation was just right for her, and soon afterwards she began seeing results. She was less stressed and happier than before. When she entered her third trimester she was much more confident and was able to write her own affirmations. They helped so much that she was relaxed during her childbirth and remained calm when she returned to work.

◎ ◎ ◎ ◎ ◎ ◎ ◎

In this chapter you learned:

1. Why use a shortcut

2. What are some common causes for stress during pregnancy

3. Positive affirmations to use during pregnancy

In the next chapter you will learn about some stress-relief complementary tools to help you implement the positive affirmation technique.

"It seems to me shallow and arrogant for any man in these times to claim he is completely self-made, that he owes all his success to his own unaided efforts. Many hands and hearts and minds generally contribute to anyone's notable achievements."

~Walt Disney (entertainer and entrepreneur)

CHAPTER 8: STRESS RELIEF COMPLEMENTARY TOOLS TO HELP IMPLEMENT THE POSITIVE AFFIRMATION TECHNIQUE

WORKING WITH STRESS

The positive affirmations technique is very powerful when it comes to dealing with stress. It's easy to use and has a very fast-acting effect, so it is very suitable for helping you throughout your pregnancy. The technique works on you mind and targets your subconscious.

Sometimes it's good to combine working on your mind with other techniques. Now that your body is changing so rapidly, it's a good idea to work on taking care of your physical body as well.

During your pregnancy you can develop habits that will last and benefit you even after your child is born, which will help both you and your baby. Working with your body will also give you a lot of confidence, especially if you struggle with worries about your weight or your looks. The strength you get from physical exercise and a good diet will also help you when it's time for your labor.

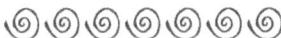

Due to a busy job and ongoing problems with her mother's health, Eleanor had a lot of stress during her pregnancy. Her doctors told her to be careful or she could develop high blood pressure. She was very concerned about her own health, especially since both she and her sick mother were overweight.

She wanted desperately to work on her mind, but whenever she tried, she'd find that it was impossible for her to relax. There was always something in the way. So she decided that she needed to work on her body before she could work on her mind.

Eleanor began a strict workout routine and set up a healthy diet for herself. Gradually she began to lose weight, feel stronger and eventually more relaxed, as her health improved. Her blood pressure went down to normal levels. When she once again tried to work with positive affirmations, Eleanor found the process to be much easier. By her third trimester she was relaxed and calm. That calmness lasted even after her baby was born, and so did her new workout routines and healthy diet.

〰️ ◎ ◎ ◎ ◎ ◎ ◎ ◎

TECHNIQUES TO RELIEVE STRESS

There are many ways to help you relax your body. Every woman is different and has her own preferences, so choose which techniques work best for you. Here are a few suggestions on what you can do.

1. Eat healthy food.

Eating the right kind of food can have a great impact on your stress levels. Some foods can boost your body's levels of serotonin, which works to calm your brain. Other foods lower your body's levels of adrenaline and cortisol: stress hormones that could damage both you and your baby.

Whole-grain breads, cereals and pastas can increase your brain's production of serotonin, a chemical that works to calm your body. This kind of food also stabilizes your blood sugar.

Oranges and other fruits rich in vitamin C strengthen your immune system. Studies have also shown that people who took vitamin C supplements before a challenging task, had their blood pressure and cortisol levels return to normal more quickly than those who didn't, showing that vitamin C can in fact lower stress.

Many women suffer from headaches and fatigue during their pregnancy, which only makes the stress worse. In fact, they might be suffering from a magnesium deficiency. Eating spinach, soybeans or green leafy vegetables can help you replenish your magnesium stores.

Fatty fish like salmon and tuna contain plenty of Omega 3 fatty acids, which can help protect you against heart diseases and depression. Nuts such as almonds, walnuts and pistachios can lower your blood pressure; they also contain a lot of healthy vitamins. Avocados and bananas contain potassium, which also lowers your blood pressure.

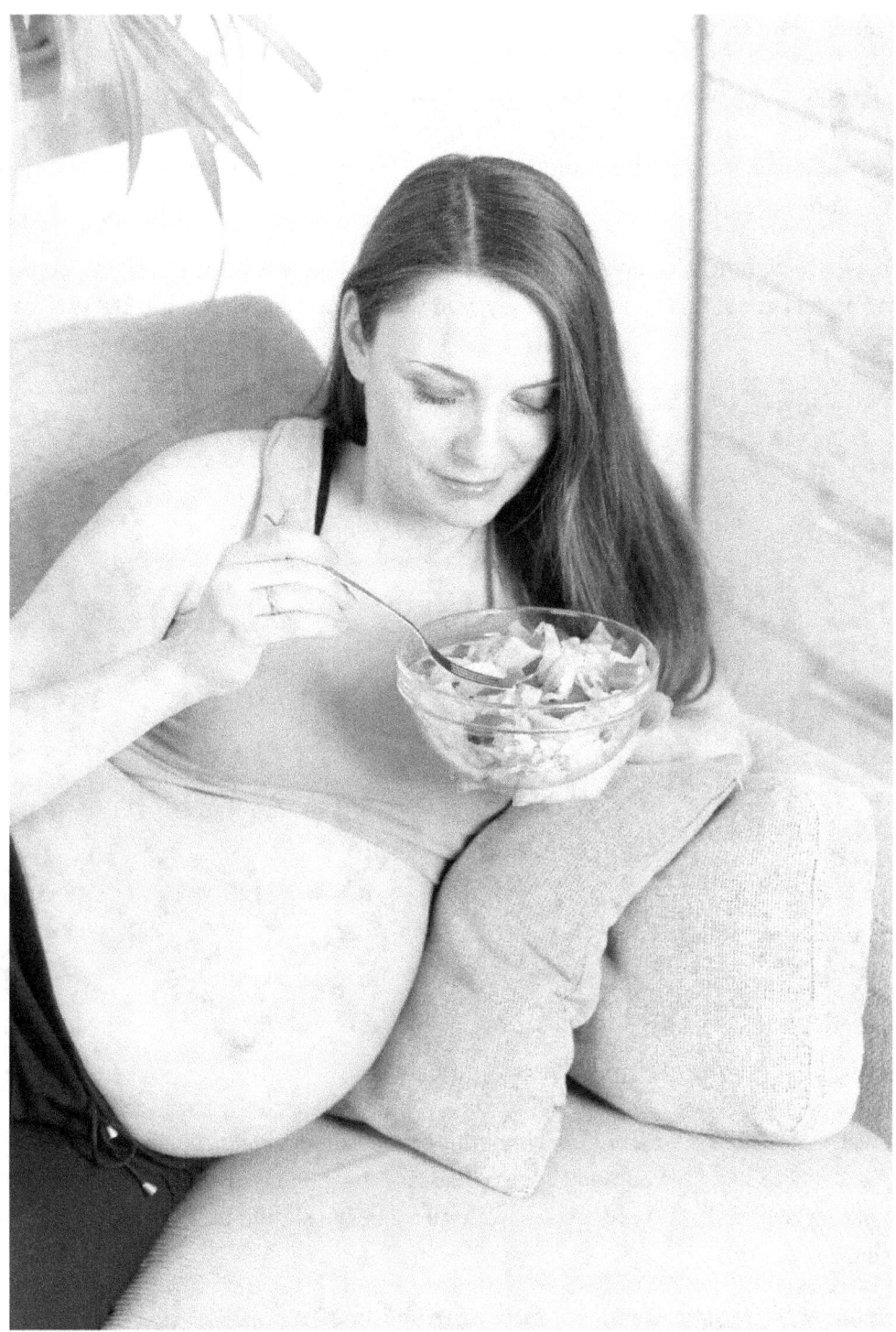

You can learn more about simple and easy tactics to prepare nourishing meals during your pregnancy in my book *Pregnancy Diet : A Practical Guide For Busy Women*

2. Practice prenatal yoga

You can combine a healthy diet with some good prenatal yoga to boost your wellbeing and lower your stress. Yoga works with both your body and mind at the same time. Studies have also shown that women who do yoga during their pregnancies, experience less pain during labor.

You may also want to pick up swimming or walking, which will relax your body as well as make you feel good. With a healthy body, you will notice how your mind starts to calm down as well.

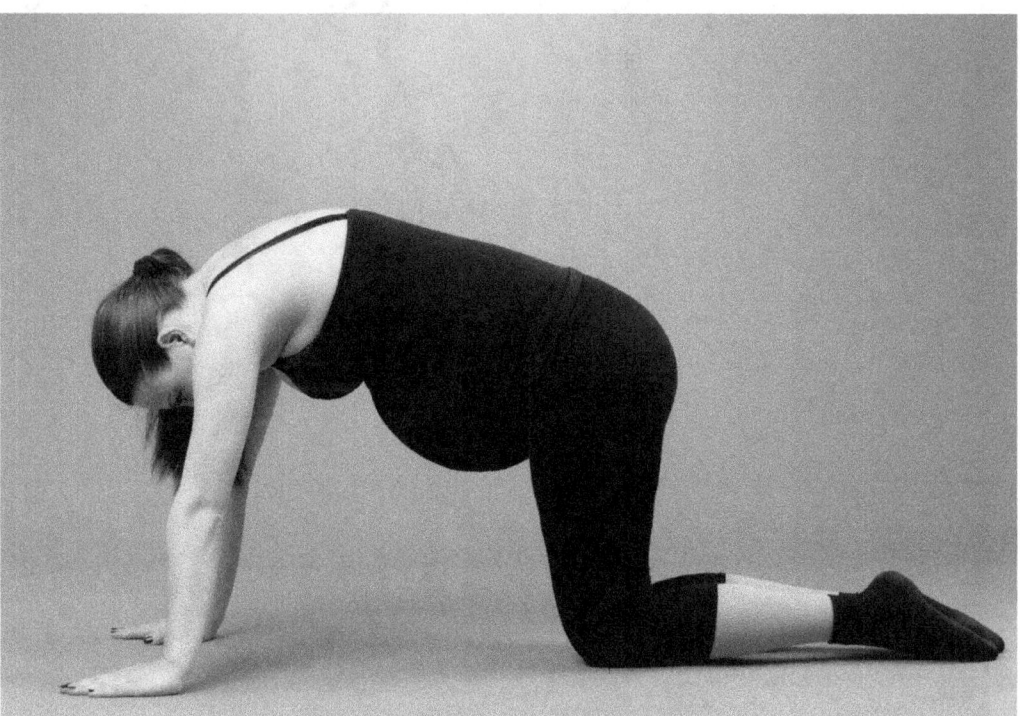

3. The Five Senses Tool

The Five Senses Tool is a technique I invented for myself during pregnancy as part of my own personal toolkit. It is named this way because our body feels and gains experiences through our five senses. In order to relax our bodies, we should first relax and calm our five senses.

The five senses are sight, hearing, touch, taste and smell.

The Five Senses Tool suggests that you need to find your strongest sense. Perhaps you are a person who sees very well and thus prefers visual influences. Perhaps your hearing or touch is very well-developed. Many women find that their senses of taste and smell improve during pregnancy.

Once you have found your dominant sense, the one you receive most influence from, you should work to inspire and calm this sense. If your strongest sense is hearing, for example, you should make a habit of listening to calm, relaxing music every day. If it is your smell, try placing sweet-smelling flowers or burn incense around the house, so you always smell something good.

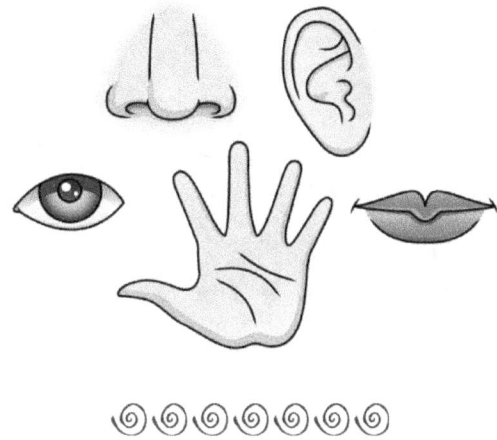

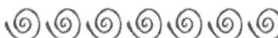

Adele wanted to work with positive affirmations during her pregnancy, but she found that her mind was too preoccupied most of the time, preventing her from doing so efficiently. She began working with her body and set forth a diet regiment, but still felt that something was missing. That's when she began working with the Five Senses Tool.

She found that her strongest sense was touch, and she began going to prenatal massage every week to calm and relax her body. Eventually she found herself in a place where she could work with the positive affirmation technique. This time the affirmations worked perfectly for her, and she reduced her stress in time for her labor. Once her child was born, she continued to use the Five Senses Tool combined with positive affirmations to stay calm throughout the stressful first years of her child.

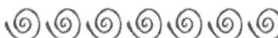

In this chapter you learned about:

1. Working with stress

2. Techniques to relieve stress

3. The Five Senses Tool

In the next chapter we will look at what we have learned so far and talk about the next step.

"How would your life be different if...you were conscious about the food you ate, the people you surround yourself with, and the media you watch, listen to, or read? Let today be the day...You pay attention to what you feed your mind, your body, and your life. Create a nourishing environment conducive to your growth and well-being today."
~Steve Maraboli (speaker and author)

CHAPTER 9: SUMMARY

Thank you for taking your time to read this book. You should now have a good understanding about the positive affirmation technique. The book has taken you step by step through the process of dealing with the stress you might experience during your pregnancy. You now have a new and easy tool to deal with stress, and I hope it will help you in the future.

It's my hope that you have by now understood the power of positive thoughts and how your thoughts can influence your subconscious. By changing our thoughts, we can change our emotional response to them and in turn, their influences on our lives. What we had learned to perceive as "stressful" or "dangerous", we can, with the use of positive affirmations, begin to see as "natural" and "empowering".

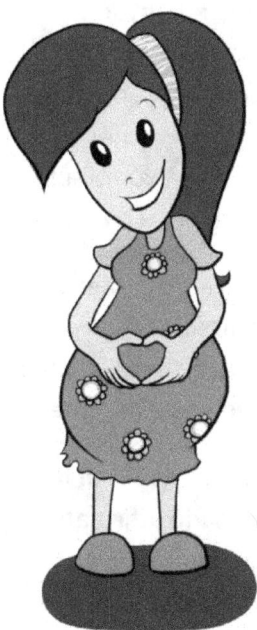

There are many reasons to feel stressed during pregnancy. You might be worried that your body will change too much and not return to normal after your childbirth. The guidelines for what you're allowed to eat or drink might cause stress in your life. All those raging hormones might be giving you a hard time and cause tension between you and your partner. We all worry about the health of our baby, but it shouldn't make you stressed. Whatever the reason is that you feel stress, you don't need to suffer.

Stress can be very harmful to both you and your baby. Many who suffer from stress go through periods of insomnia, and now more than ever you need those full nights of sleep. Stress can increase your blood pressure, which can put you at risk for strokes or heart attacks while pregnant.

Stress can also transfer to your baby. Constricted blood vessels due to stress might not allow enough nutrients to pass to your child. Stress hormones have been linked to premature labor and even miscarriages. It is therefore urgent that you deal with your stress and take care of yourself.

Fortunately for you, there's a simple and efficient tool in positive affirmations. By writing your own affirmation, you create a personal statement that will reprogram your subconscious. If you worry about not being able to lose weight during pregnancy, you can reduce your stress and remove your worries by letting yourself know, many times a day that you are beautiful. Concern about your baby's health can be replaced with confidence in the fact that he is healthy and happy.

Using positive affirmations requires a lot of repetition. Only by constant repetition can your positive affirmation become embedded in your subconscious and have an effect on your state of mind. It's therefore crucial that you practice every day. These few minutes of working with affirmations can give you a lifetime of stress-free joy and health.

Many women, for whatever reasons are not able to write their own affirmations, and for them I put together a list of pre-made affirmations to use. By thinking about what worries you the most (in regards to pregnancy, childbirth or your baby), you can find a pre-made affirmation that will fit your needs.

Most people benefit from using a combination of techniques to deal with stress. If you find that working with affirmations is hard, you might want to consider working with your body first. Eating healthy can reduce the levels of stress hormones in your body and give you the energy you need to go through your pregnancy successfully. Practicing prenatal yoga or swimming can further increase your energy and give you strength for the upcoming childbirth. You can also work with calming your five senses and thereby becoming more relaxed in your daily life. Combined with the positive affirmations technique, these are all very powerful tools to use for stress reduction.

THE ROAD FROM HERE

During the course of this book you have been made to think about what creates stress in your life. You have also been given instructions for how to create your own positive affirmations and how these should be used.

Now, it's time to practice. No one is perfect from the outset, and we all need time to make changes in our lives. By practicing and repeating your positive affirmations several times every day, you make them a part of your daily routine. In time, these affirmations will become part of your subconscious; that's when they will begin reducing your stress most effectively.

You now have a tool to help you pass through this challenging time without unnecessary stress. Worrying is completely normal, but you can now face those worries with a confident, strong mind. You will be tranquil, peaceful and full of faith in yourself. When the time comes for your labor, you will believe in your own ability to give birth and that you can make it natural, happy and healthy for both you and your baby.

All you have to do is take action. Print your positive affirmations and hang them somewhere you can see them. This will help you remember to implement them effectively. Repeat them every day, as often as you can. For every day you don't take action, you and your baby might suffer unnecessarily from stress. So start today.

I wish you a good, peaceful pregnancy and an easy birth.

"When you swim you don't grab hold of the water, because if you do, you will sink and drown. Instead you relax, and float."

~Alan Watts (philosopher)

Bonus Chapter - How to strengthen your mind

As we have seen in this book, the image visualization technique is a valuable tool designed to influence and strengthen your mind.

Our mind is our most powerful tool when it comes to dealing with stress, anxiety and fear. Using only our mind, we can turn a negative outlook into a positive one and rid ourselves of worries. The problem is, most often we don't know how to use our minds to the fullest extent. Only when we learn to do so, can we enjoy the benefits of a strong, confident mind.

Our minds are constantly influenced by what we see, hear and read every day. Some people let every impression enter straight into their minds, and some know how to sort between what is good and what is bad for them. The difference between these people is their awareness of how things influence them.

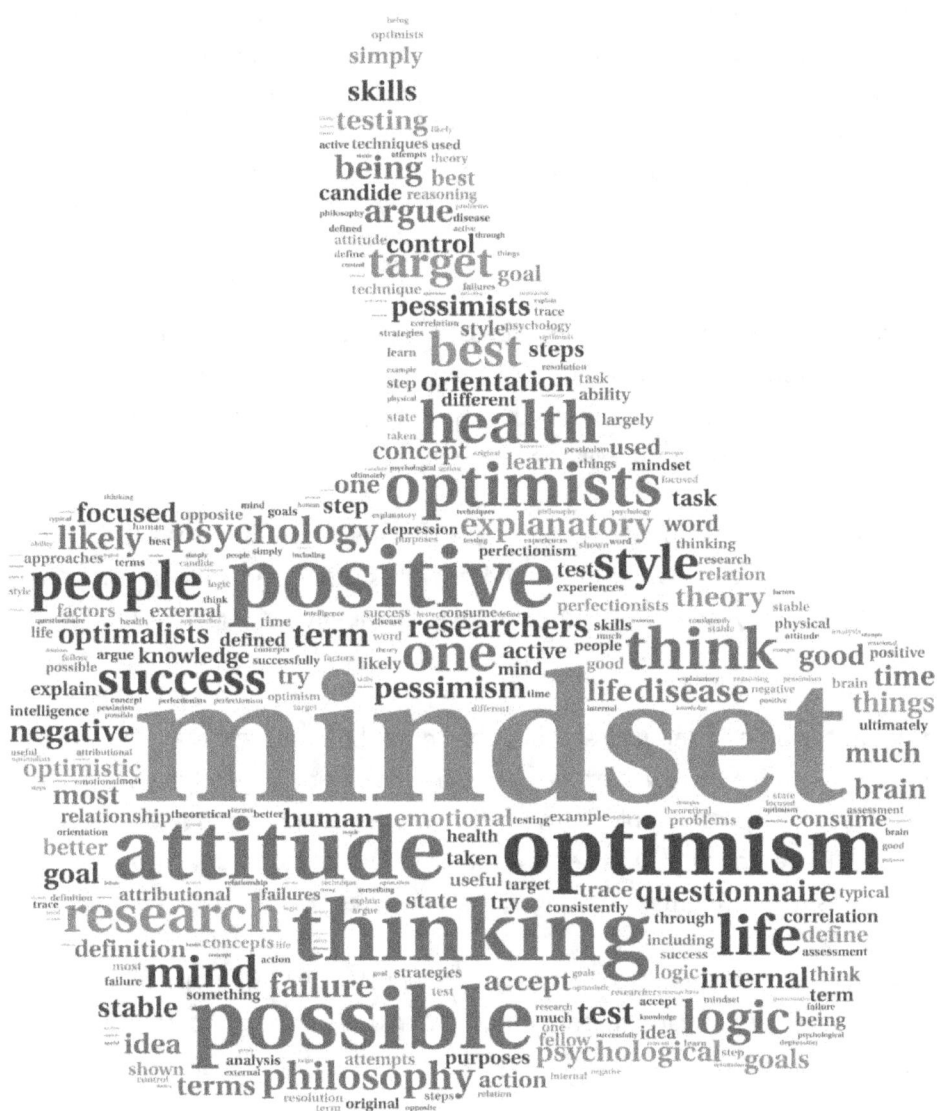

Mariah came into contact with people who told of frightening tales of pregnancy and childbirth, every day, while she was working at a hospital. Women told her what had gone wrong and how painful labor was. When Mariah became pregnant with her first child, she found those stories difficult to ignore. The result was a stressful pregnancy because she worried every day that something would go wrong.

During labor, Mariah was terrified about the pain and became very tense. The result was that her contractions were much more painful than necessary. Only after a while did she realize that the pain wasn't as bad throughout her pregnancy as she had thought it would be. She began to relax and found that she didn't need to worry about it as much. In the end, she had a fast and uncomplicated delivery of a healthy baby boy.

ⓢ ⓢ ⓢ ⓢ ⓢ ⓢ ⓢ

Worry brings unnecessary stress and tension. You can rid yourself of all of this by learning more about the powerful tools that will help you strengthen your mind. Minimize bad influences and expose your mind to positive images. The more you can control your mind, the easier it will be to get what you want.

After a healthy pregnancy and a natural birth of my first child, I realized that I owed much of my success to the way I managed my mind. I decided to learn more about the mind, which is a very powerful tool, and use my newly-acquired technique on other aspects of my life.

During my quest of learning more about the mind, I encountered a great mentor, Bob Proctor. Bob is a talented speaker who teaches professional coaching seminars and his work focuses on helping people harness the power of their mind to succeed in their lives. He is also a teaching master of the Law of Attraction, which stipulates that focusing on positive thoughts can bring a positive outcome.

I had participated in a number of his seminars which were the start of a big change in my life. The most important lesson for me was **that repetition is important when talking about the mind**.

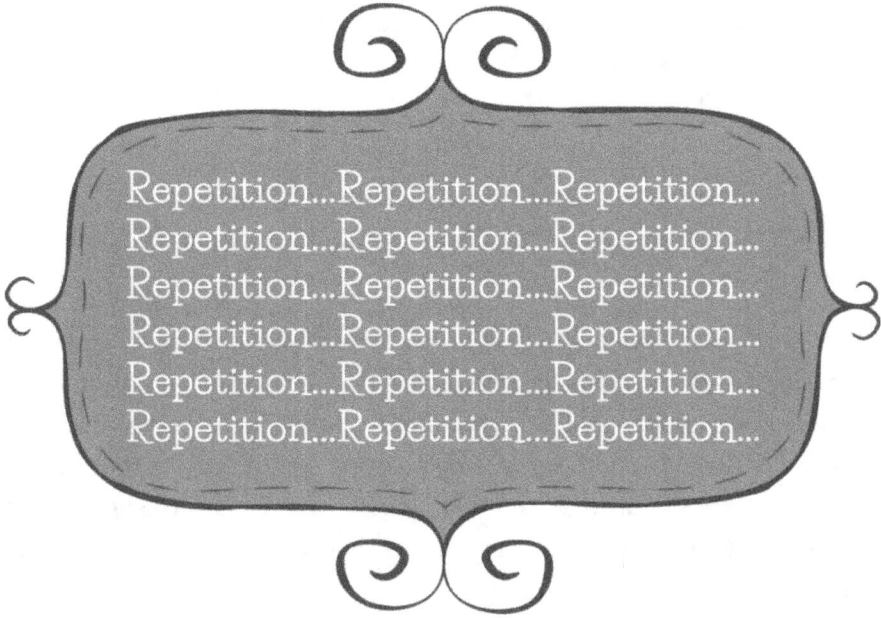

Repetition can be done in several ways:

1. Listen to audio lessons while driving in your car or doing exercises, etc. I made it a habit to listen to one lesson, every day. Usually I listened to each lesson 30 days in a row in order for it to sink into my mind and become a part of it.

An audio which I can greatly recommend is "The Strangest Secret" by Earl Nightingale. This is one of the most influential messages on audio, and it explores the question of what it takes to succeed in the ever-changing world of today.

2. Get a positive insight every day. This is a powerful tool to grow your own awareness and learn more about your mind. I like to open my day with "Insight of the Day" by Bob Proctor. By signing up for a daily insight, you will receive a short message that will give you something positive to focus on.

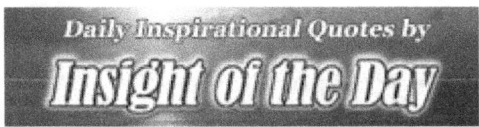

3. Participate in weekly sessions of learning new information about the mind. I signed up for Bob's streaming club. In this club I have the opportunity to meet him once a week, to

learn the most efficient and valuable lessons about the mind. I've found that attending the weekly meetings is like going to a "mind gym."

◎ ◎ ◎ ◎ ◎ ◎ ◎

My friend Sophia had a difficult first pregnancy and suffered from a wide variety of symptoms as well as post-partum depression. When she became pregnant with her second child, she was determined to change her mindset and have a positive experience during pregnancy and childbirth. She signed up for Bob Proctor's daily insight, attended his weekly seminars and listened to every audio book on the subject that she could find, while driving to work every day. When it was time for her childbirth she felt relaxed and at ease. The delivery went very well, without complications, and this time around, she didn't suffer from depression.

◎ ◎ ◎ ◎ ◎ ◎ ◎

I hope you will find these tools helpful and that you now know where to begin in your quest to expand your mind and to find more positive influences. This will help you throughout the challenging time that is pregnancy and childbirth. Afterwards, you and your baby will be able to reap the benefits of your training, since you will have a more positive outlook and a strong mind, free from negative thoughts and unnecessary worries.

"You are today where your thoughts have brought you; you will be tomorrow where your thoughts take you."

-James Lane Allen (author)

You can find more helpful tools in my other books:

Childbirth without Fear: Using the Image Visualization Technique to Conquer Your Fears

SPECIAL BONUS - THE TREE OF POWER

Throughout this book you learned about the importance of positive affirmations in order to create a stress-free environment for yourself. I believe that you will have more tools in your kit than this one.

There are many ways you can reduce your stress during pregnancy. Many women find that walking or swimming makes them calm. Others use the Image Visualization Technique, which focuses on using images rather than words, to reprogram your subconscious. You can use vision boards very effectively together with your positive affirmations.

Eating healthy is very important for a happy and stress-free pregnancy. Reading up on what lies ahead might give you some peace of mind if you fear the uncertainty about pregnancy and childbirth. Taking a prenatal course can teach you many valuable tools and also put you in contact with other moms-to-be who might share your worries.

Don't forget to keep your sense of humor and to stay close with your partner during this time.

I created the Power Tree especially for women like you, so you can print it and write down all the positive assets and tools you have to prepare you for the upcoming labor. Hang it in front of you and make sure you look at it every day. Put a copy of it in your "birth bag" so that you can draw your strength from it.

Attached is a sample of my Power Tree:

My Pregnancy Tree of Power

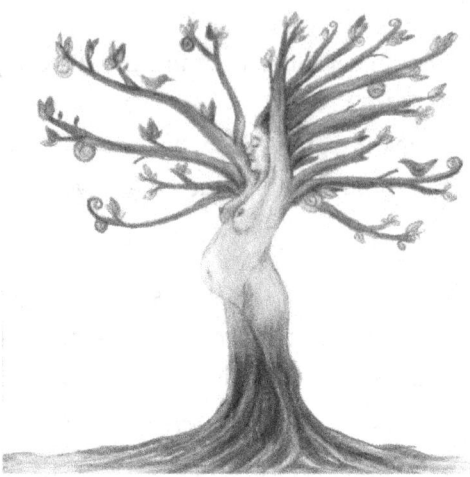

My positive assets and tools that I have for my upcoming childbirth

1. Weekly exercise of prenatal yoga

2. Practice breathing techniques

3. Cope with my childbirth fears with the Image visualization technique & the Positive affirmations technique

4. Perform a perineum massage by my partner

5. Maintaining a well-balanced diet

6. Acupuncture treatments once a month

Scan the code below to download your free copy of the your tree of power .

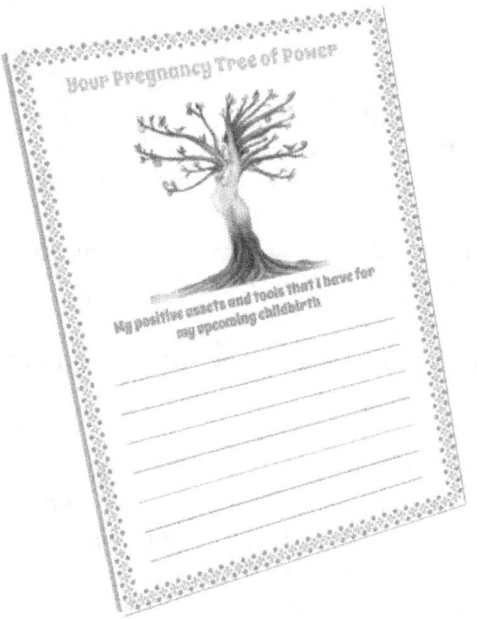

I wish you a happy pregnancy and childbirth.

I hope you have enjoyed this book and now feel that you have an additional tool in your kit when the time comes for your labor. I wish you a relaxed, natural and calm birth.

ABOUT THE AUTHOR

Einat is a mother to a lovely girl.
She has been studying for the last 15 years the powerful ways to use your mind & subconscious and live a quiet, peaceful and better life.
She tries to live according to the methods she's learned in all areas of her life.

Einat believes in the principles of flow , liberation and positive thinking.
That's why she loves the shape of the spiral.
She implements these principles in her daily life.
She's on an endless journey of her personal development and tries to do the best she can.

When she became pregnant with her first daughter, she implemented the tools she learned about herself in order to have an easy, pleasant and empowering pregnancy. Einat had many concerns about the birth process but with the tools and techniques which she applied to herself she was able to overcome these concerns and gave a natural childbirth to a healthy daughter.

Einat is the co-founder of a new pregnancy web site www.myPregnancyToolkit.com that brings a set of practical tools for pregnant women that focuses on the pregnancy issues from the mind's perspective.

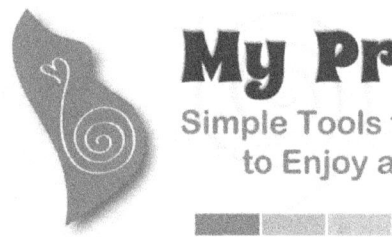

My Pregnancy Toolkit
Simple Tools for Busy Women that will Enable You to Enjoy an Easy Pregnancy and Childbirth

MORE BOOKS AND PRODUCTS BY THE AUTHOR

Childbirth without Fear: Using the Image Visualization Technique to Conquer Your Fears

In this book you will learn about the image visualization technique and how it can help you eliminate your upcoming childbirth fears. It will help you reduce your stress and you'll even begin to enjoy your pregnancy. This technique can effectively replace your fearful mental images of childbirth with those that are reinforcing and positive.

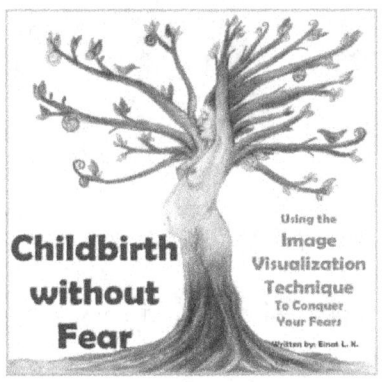

Childbirth without Fear - Guided Meditations to help you Conquer Your Fears

The *audio guided meditations* are part of a set of helpful tools that can help you eliminate your upcoming childbirth fears. These meditations can serve as a stand alone tool and also as a complement to the book *Childbirth without Fear: Using the Image Visualization Technique to Conquer Your Fears*. They are easy to practice and can be used any time and anywhere.

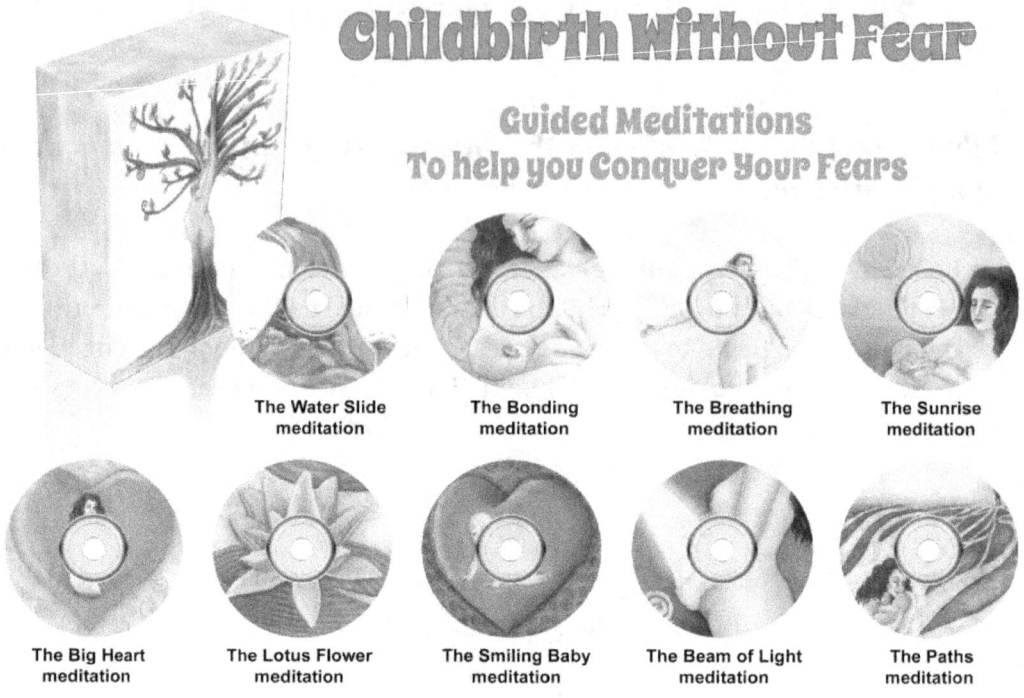

Pregnancy Diet: A Practical Guide for Busy Women

In this book you will learn about simple and easy tactics for preparing nourishing meals during your pregnancy, so that you and your baby can enjoy a healthy pregnancy.

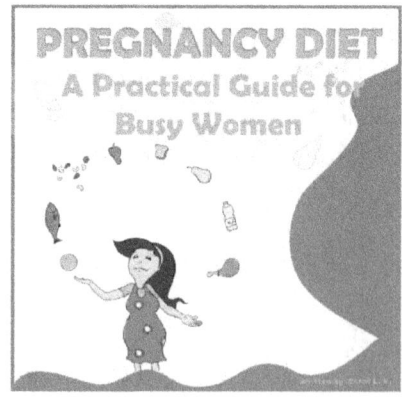

www.ingramcontent.com/pod-product-compliance
Lightning Source LLC
Chambersburg PA
CBHW081244280526
45787CB00006B/2790